Flexible Dieting
&
IIFYM

*How to Burn Fat & Build Muscle by
Eating Your Favorite Foods*

The author of this book has taken careful measures to share vital information about the subject. May its readers acquire the right knowledge, wisdom, inspiration, and therefore succeed.

Table of Contents

Introduction

Congratulations on downloading this book and thank you for doing so.

The following chapters will teach you everything that you need to know about Flexible Dieting and IIFYM (If It Fits Your Macros) approach.

Chapter 1 discusses the basics, so that you will have a better understanding of Flexible Dieting and the IIFYM approach. You will learn the macronutrients, which are essential to any healthy diet, as well as how to calculate the number of calories that your body needs, among others.

Chapter 2 talks about weight loss. Learn how you can effectively lose weight, the importance of calorie deficit to weight loss, and others. If losing weight is your primary purpose for going on a diet, then you should not miss this chapter.

Chapter 3 reveals the fad diets. It is good to know these fad diets, so you will not fall for their traps and scams. By knowing the fad diets, you will also understand the diets that work, and why Flexible Dieting grounded on the IIFYM approach is an effective diet program.

Chapter 4 lays down effective exercises that will allow you to burn more calories and sculpt a better-looking physique. Diet alone is not enough. If you want to be truly healthy, you must also look healthy — and the way to achieve this is by combining a healthy diet with regular exercise.

Chapter 5 shows the keys to success. These are the best practices that you should observe which can further guarantee your success. Regardless of whether you follow the Flexible Diet program or any other healthy diet plans, these keys to success will give you helpful tips and tricks that you need to have a healthy and fit body.

Chapter 6 discusses the common pitfalls that you should avoid. These are the mistakes and blunders that those who start out on a diet usually face. It is best that you are aware of these pitfalls, so that you can make the necessary adjustments and not commit the same mistakes.

There are plenty of books on this subject on the market, thanks again for choosing this one! Every effort was made to ensure it is full of as much useful information as possible. Please enjoy!

Chapter 1: The Basics

Flexible Dieting, also referred to as IIFYM (If It Fits Your Macros), is one of the best diet programs in the world. If you are tired of following a strict diet plan, if you want a diet that you can safely turn into a lifestyle, then Flexible Dieting is the one for you.

Understanding Flexible Dieting

As the name already implies, it is flexible in the sense that this diet program allows you to consume even not so nutritious foods from time to time. Hence, it has the benefit of allowing you to eat your favorite pizza or ice cream. Yes, you do not have to shy away from sweets. After all, they are delicious! With Flexible Dieting, you can become fit and healthy while enjoying various delicious foods, even the not so nutritious ones. It is a well-balanced diet that focuses on your macros by using the IIFYM approach. By keeping within the recommended macros level for your body, you can get fit and healthy. After all, dieting should not be a sad experience. It is supposed to be a way of life.

The Macronutrients

The body needs nourishment to sustain life. Inside the body, there are different parts that engage in important activities which require nutrients. Even as people sit still or sleep, the cells in the body are continuously moving and changing to maintain, repair or grow tissues. There is a need to constantly replenish the nutrients and energy the body uses so that its different parts can continue to function normally.

The organic compounds: carbohydrates, fat, and proteins, are the nutrients the body needs in big amounts; hence, they are called macronutrients. These nutrients provide energy, and the energies released from them are measured in calories.

The number of calories, or energy, a food has depends on how much carbohydrates, fats, and proteins the food contains. When completely metabolized in the body, 1 gram of carbohydrate yields 4 calories; 1 gram of protein yields 4 calories; and 1 gram of fat yields 9 calories.

These macronutrients do not only provide energy for the body, but they are essential for other bodily functions. Let us take a closer look at each of these macronutrients:

Carbohydrates

Many people mistakenly avoid carbohydrates because they think these are fattening. Well, this is true for candies, soft drinks, and other sweets. But, avoiding carbohydrates like wheat, legumes, and vegetables, would be detrimental to health.

Almost all cell activities depend on glucose for energy, especially the brain and nerve cells. Without adequate glucose, the body is forced to make energy from protein, primarily protein from liver and skeletal muscles.

Having fewer carbohydrates also makes the brain rely on fat to get energy. Fat, when metabolized, will form ketone bodies during starvation. This will actually help you lose weight as your body undergoes ketosis. But, in the long run, ketosis will disturb the acid-base balance of your blood because of the acidic nature of ketone bodies.

To prevent using body protein and ketosis, adequate intake of carbohydrates is needed. At least 50 to 100 grams carbohydrates a day from good carbohydrate sources is recommended.

Also, including healthy sources of carbohydrates in your diet provides your body with soluble and insoluble fibers. These fibers can help you maintain or lose weight, fight heart diseases and prevent constipation and other digestive ailments.

With these benefits provided by sources of carbohydrates, aside from the phytochemicals, vitamins, and minerals you can get, carbohydrates are important to maintain a good health. You just need to be wise in selecting carbohydrates that are rich in fiber and low in sugar.

Protein

Protein plays a vital role in the body. It is the building block of not only muscles, but also of blood, skin, and most parts of the body. For example, the protein, collagen, is needed as a matrix in the formation of teeth, tendons, and ligaments. Also, it gives strength to the cells of the artery walls to withstand the pressure of blood flowing through them and much more. Protein is the material used in all these things, so protein is needed to maintain and replace the damaged cells. You need protein for your hair, to synthesize nails, and your muscles need new protein to grow larger and strengthen them in response to exercise. For example, if you engage in weight training and only consume a small amount of protein, you cannot expect for your muscles to grow and increase in size. This is because muscle growth depends not only on the exercises that you do; you also need to consume adequate amounts of protein for your body.

Protein is also used to make enzymes to aid in digestion; hormones to facilitate the different mechanisms in the body, like insulin that regulates blood glucose; and antibodies to defend the body against diseases.

Protein also helps maintain the fluid balance of the body. Sufficient protein in the cells helps the tissues to not accumulate excess fluids and not to swell. This results in high productivity levels of transporting nutrients and oxygen to cells and the removal of wastes in the cells.

Protein has the ability to donate and accept hydrogen ions. With this capability, protein acts as a buffer to maintain the acid-base balance of the body. As a result, alkalosis and acidosis of the blood is prevented.

If there is not enough glucose in the blood, the protein in the muscles can be broken down and be converted to glucose. In this, the level of glucose in the blood can be maintained.

These are only some functions of protein in the body. There are still many activities that protein plays an integral part of. For these reasons, protein-rich foods must be given importance in the diet. But it does not necessarily mean that you should consume protein in excess. Overeating protein-rich foods, especially from an animal source, can be a great threat to your health. Moderation and a combination of high-quality protein from animal sources, and low-quality protein from plants are crucial for proper protein nutrition. For vegetarians to improve their protein intake, they often consume a variety of grains, legumes, nuts, seeds, and vegetables.

Fat

People perceive fat as something bad for their health. It is a common misconception to avoid fat thoroughly to improve health and lose weight. But fat is only damaging to your health if you consume too much of some of its types.

Fat is a nutrient that needs to be included moderately in your diet. It not only functions as our stored energy, it can also cushion the bones and organs in the body against shock and it can protect the body from extreme temperatures.

Fats, specifically the phospholipids, are part of the cellular membrane. They can easily allow fat-soluble nutrients, like vitamins and hormones, to go in and out of cells.

Another role of fats is synthesizing bile, sex hormones and vitamin D from cholesterol in the body. So, cholesterol is not really bad because about 800 to 1500 mg cholesterol a day is converted by the liver to these compounds. Cholesterol will only be harmful if it accumulates on the artery walls and forms plaques. This may lead to atherosclerosis.

Essential fatty acids, Omega-3 and Omega-6, are needed for brain development, growth, and they are necessary to prevent and treat heart diseases. Fat, like carbohydrates and protein, is important in maintaining good health. It does not need to be avoided at all. Moderation in taking the right kind of fat, like the monounsaturated and polyunsaturated fats from plants and fish, and limiting the consumption of saturated fats and trans-fat are considerations to achieve good health.

Energy needs

Having enough energy to maintain a healthy and active lifestyle is a must. Too much energy can lead to being overweight and too little can lead to being undernourished. How many calories you need depends on three factors:
1. Physical activity.
2. Thermic effect of food.
3. Basal metabolism or resting energy expenditure.

Growth, pregnancy and lactation are other factors that can influence your calorie needs. These need additional energy.

Physical activity

Physical activity contributes about 20% to 30% to calorie expenditure. The intensity, duration, and frequency of the physical activity can greatly influence how many calories will be used up. If the calories consumed were used up by exercise or another activity, the body can maintain or lose weight.

Thermic Effect of Food

Thermic Effect of Food, also known as Dietary Induced Thermogenesis or Specific Dynamic Action, indicates the amount of energy used in digesting, absorbing and metabolizing food plus the basal metabolism rate in consideration of the effect of the chemicals found in foods.

Basal metabolic rate

The body, even at rest, expends energy to sustain involuntary activities, like circulation, digestion and respiration, among others.
The basal metabolism is responsible for using up to 70% of

total calories. Although the BMR varies according to different factors:

a. Age. As you age, your BMR decreases.

b. Sex. Because of difference in body mass and hormones, women have lower BMR, about 6-10%, than males.

c. Body size/shape. How tall and the shape of your body influence your BMR. A tall and willowy woman will have a higher BMR than a petite woman.

d. Body temperature. Normal temperature does not really affect BMR. But if you have a fever or if you are shivering because of a very low temperature, your BMR will increase in response.

e. Growth. If you are still growing, your body is building up lots of tissues, therefore BMR is high.

f. State of body condition. People who are obese, malnourished or have hypothyroidism have low BMR. While people who are active, have menstruation or have hyperthyroidism, etc. have higher BMR.

g. Sleep. BMR is decreased by about 10% during sleeping because of the relaxation of muscles.

h. Diet. Abruptly reducing your calorie intake in high level or starving yourself can greatly decrease your BMR.

i. Hormones. Hormones secreted by the pituitary glands and adrenals can affect metabolism but to a lesser degree.

j. Genetics. Some people are blessed with good metabolism since they were born. They can easily burn up the calories they have consumed even without exerting much effort.

k. External Temperature. Cold temperature in the environment and prolonged exposure to hot temperature can increase BMR.

Steps in calculating your diet

1. Calculate your desirable body weight. There are many methods to estimate your DBW and one of them is the BMI Based.

$$DBW = (meter)^2 \times 21 \text{ for women}$$

$$\times 22 \text{ for men}$$

For example:

An adult sedentary female who stands at 1.76 m

$$DBW = (1.76)^2 \times 21$$
$$= 65.05 \text{ kg or } 65 \text{ kg}$$

2. Determine the reasonable calorie allowance by multiplying the DBW with the following values according to:

Activity	Kcal/kg DBW/day
Bed rest but mobile	27.5
Sedentary (office clerk, secretary, cashier, etc.)	30.0
Light (driver, nurse, teacher, tailor, etc.)	
Moderate (carpenter, painter, heavy housework, etc.)	35.0
Very active (athlete, lumberman, etc.)	40.0
	45.0

For example:
Total Energy Allowance of a sedentary female with a desirable body weight of 65 kg
= 65 x 30 = 1950 kcal

3. Determine the carbohydrate, protein and fat by:
Percentage Distribution:

Carbohydrates - 45 to 65 % of TEA
Protein   - 10 to 35% of TEA
Fat   - 20 to 35% of TEA

The distribution will depend on your diet prescription or usual food habits.
For example (using the TEA of the sedentary female with a DBW of 65 kg):
For a normal diet, 65% of the TEA can be allotted for carbohydrates, 15% protein and 20% of TEA for fat. The equivalent of the energy distributions of these macronutrients are:

Carbohydrates   - 1950 x 0.65 = 1267.5 kcal
Protein   - 1950 x 0.15 = 292.5 kcal
Fat   - 1950 x 0.20 = 390 kcal

After this, calculate how many grams of carbohydrates, protein and fat you can have by dividing the calories for each nutrient by the physiological value. Remember, there are 4 kcal in every gram of carbohydrates and protein and 9 kcal for every gram of fat.

Carbohydrates: 1267.5/ 4 = 316.88 g or 315 g
Protein: 292.5/4   = 73.13 g or 75 g
Fat: 390/9   = 43.33 g or 45 g

For ease, you can round off calories to the nearest 50, and round off the macronutrients to the nearest 5 grams.

4. With the values you've got, you can plan a healthy diet that can suit your needs. If you want to lose weight, subtract 500 kcal from your TEA. 1lb can be deducted to your weight every week; and if you add exercise to your diet, you can lose another pound, a total of 2lbs per week.

Planning a healthy diet

The body needs proper nourishment to support the many activities happening inside. So, proper food selection must be observed to achieve good health and avoid weight gain. Here are some guidelines that can be observed in food selection:

Adequacy

In planning a diet, make sure you are able to receive ample essential nutrients, fiber and energy that your body needs to maintain good health.

Some nutrients can be synthesized in the body but there are some that should be only supplied by food. For example, calcium is not only stored in the bones, it is also constantly used by the body to make hormones, enzymes, etc. Calcium in the body depletes and if not replaced, it can have a detrimental effect on health. To avoid deficiency, make sure to select foods that can sufficiently provide calcium and other nutrients that the body needs.

Balance

A balanced diet means consuming each type of food in proportion to what the body needs. Eating enough and not too much of each kind of food is key. Balanced meals have a good proportion of carbohydrates, protein and fat.

Moderation

Eating foods rich in sugar and fat gives pleasure to most people. But eating them in excess can result in weight gain. To avoid this, you should always remember to have these in moderation and just occasionally. Regularly eat food low in sodium, sugar and saturated fat

Energy Control

To maintain weight or lose weight, make sure to design a meal that can adequately provide energy and nutrients to your body. The amount of energy consumed must be balanced with the amount of energy required for basal metabolism and physical activities.

Nutrient density foods vs. Empty-calorie foods

Selecting foods that are nutrient dense or foods that have the most nutrients but give the least calories is a good way to avoid over consumption of energy. For example, a teaspoon of sugar and a teaspoon of honey provide the same energy, but you can get vitamins and minerals from honey. A person choosing honey to flavor a tea over sugar can meet daily nutrient needs and get lower calories. This action can promote good health.

Empty-calorie foods are foods that have low nutrients but give off a high amount of calories. Examples are potato chips, sweets, colas, etc. Energy from these foods comes mostly from sugar and fat. There is little or no energy coming from protein. Vitamins and minerals are also seldom provided.

Knowing which foods may cause more harm than benefit is a good way to plan a healthy diet. To do this, it is good to check the overall nutrient composition of foods.

Variety

Variety is another key to achieving optimum nutrition. It is not good to eat the same kind of food each day for various reasons:

a. Different foods within the same groups have different vitamins and nutrients. Example from the fruit group is citrus fruits and papaya. Citrus fruits are rich in vitamin C while papaya is rich in vitamin A. Variety of foods ensures adequacy of nutrients.

b. Some foods have substances that, when taken in excess, are harmful to health. For example spinach. Spinach has high oxalates that can lead to the formation of kidney stones. By alternating food choices, a person can minimize ingesting unwanted substances.

c. Eating the same food over and over can get boring. By changing ingredients and recipes regularly, you can ensure that your meal is always interesting.

Main Recommendations of The Dietary Guidelines for Americans, 2010

- Manage weight by controlling your calories
- Improve your physical activities and eating habits to avoid weight gain
- Consume fewer calories from foods and beverages if you are overweight
- Move your body more and lessen time spent sitting
- Observe total energy allowance during each stage of life

What you need to reduce:

- Sodium intake must be reduced to less than 2300 mg every day and reduce it further to 1500 mg a day if you are 51 years or older or have diabetes, hypertension or chronic kidney diseases
- Eat less than 10% of calories from saturated fats. Consume calories from monounsaturated and

polyunsaturated fats
- Limit trans-fat by avoiding partially hydrogenated fats and solid fats
- Do not eat much food with added sugars
- Limit your consumption of foods with refined grains
- Alcohol consumption must be in moderation

What you need to increase:
- Eat more variety of vegetables and fruits
- Consume whole grains more than refined grains
- Increase intake of low-fat or nonfat milk and milk products, or fortified soy beverages
- Choose a variety of protein-rich foods like lean meats, poultry, seafood, beans, soy products, peas, nuts and seeds
- Increase your seafood consumption by replacing meats and poultry
- Use oils more than solid fats
- Choose foods rich in potassium, fiber, calcium and vitamin D

Make healthy eating habits:
- Choose an eating pattern that can fulfill your nutrient needs and is appropriate for your calorie allowance
- Record your foods and beverages intake and consider their effect on your eating pattern
- Ensure the safety of your food to avoid foodborne illnesses by following the recommended procedures in preparing and holding your food

Chapter 2: Weight Loss

Most people who are looking for a good and effective diet program are usually looking for a way to lose weight. Of course, weight loss can be achieved through Flexible Dieting and IIFYM approach. As already discussed, you need to eat fewer calories than what your body uses in order to lose weight.

Causes of Overweight and Obesity

There are various reasons why people accumulate fat and gain weight. Most of the time, it is because they tend to take in more calories than they expend. However, there are also factors that should be considered, such as cultural, social, behavioral and others. Here is a list of causes for why people become overweight.

Genetics

Genetics play a big role with the body's response to diet and eating habits. Genetics influence how the food is metabolized in the body and how the energy that you get from food is spent. On comparable calorie intake, some people can more easily gain weight than others. The genetics of a person can also be the cause of excessive eating and massive obesity.

There are researches conducted that support claims that the genetic makeup of people affects that person's health. Researchers continuously study genomes and the proteins that affect human's body weight. Here are some proteins that greatly affect appetite control, regulation of calories and development of obesity.

Leptin

It is a protein produced by fat cells that signal the brain to suppress appetite and expend energy. It is also released by stomach cells when there is a presence of food. This protein, which acts as a hormone, plays a big role in energy balance. It can influence the rate at which a person can lose fat: the higher number of leptin in the body, the higher chance to lose fat. If the body has low levels of leptin, a person has a tendency to overeat and not burn energy.

The amount of leptin in the body is influenced by BMI. As BMI increases, leptin levels also increase. Leptin levels are also affected by consumption of fructose. Having excess fructose in the body can stimulate leptin resistance and build up fat storage.

Adiponectin

Adiponectin is another protein produced by adipose tissues that works like leptin. Its levels are affected by body fat. The less body fat you have, the more adiponectin you have.

This protein can stop inflammation and insulin resistance. With these abilities, this protein is beneficial to people with type 2 diabetes and heart diseases; the diseases obese people are prone to.

Ghrelin

This is a protein produced by stomach cells that stimulate appetite and decreases burning of calories. This goes up whenever you are on a very low-calorie diet; a reason why maintaining weight loss is difficult. Lack of sleep also increases this protein and decreases leptin but exercise helps lower ghrelin.

These proteins produced in the body are dependent on a person's genetic make-up. They are involved in energy metabolism and affect the storing or spending of energy. But with vigorous exercise and well-planned diet, a person can influence the production of these proteins and minimize the impact of genes on a person's body.

Environment and Eating Behavior

The environment greatly influences a person's attitude towards food. It can push people to fatness or thinness. The people around you and the circumstances you encounter every day are part of your environment. When you are surrounded by people who tend to eat a lot, there is big chance you will also eat a lot.

Nowadays, the environment is full of foods that are very high in calories, high in fat, inexpensively priced and taste good. However, they are also low in nutrients. They are readily available and accessible thanks to convenience stores and fast food restaurants. The competition is very high. Fast food restaurants make big portions at low prices to lure people to buy from them. So, people unconsciously consume more than they need. An increase in the rate of overweight and obese people is observed over time.

Also, the environment now requires less physical activities due to modern technology. In the malls, there are escalators and elevators. There are automobiles to use to go to places. There is little effort needed to do things because of technology. Even at home, there are televisions, computers and cellphones that contribute to the sedentary life of people.

Having a sedentary lifestyle contributes to weight gain because you do not expend much energy beyond your basal metabolic rate. Vigorous activities outside are also replaced by watching television or playing video games. And there is a big chance for you to be influenced and purchase high-calorie foods due to the advertisements you see.

There are many causes of being overweight. It can be overeating, lack of physical activity, genetics and/or a combination of all them. You can, however, still be in control of your health and weight if you choose to.

Weight-loss Strategies

When you plan your weight loss strategy, make sure you have reasonable expectations to minimize frustrations and failures. With your moderate goals, you can easily achieve or even exceed them. Consequently, you will be more motivated to continue.

A reasonable weight loss of ½ to 2 pounds a week or 10% of body weight over six months can be expected. This gradual weight loss is most likely to be maintained than abrupt weight loss using fad diets.

Keep in mind that losing weight and having a healthy body is a lifelong journey. To be successful in weight management, you need to make eating healthy and doing physical activities part of your daily life. Here are some recommendations to help you.

Develop good eating plans

In making your menu plans, you need to consider foods that you like, that are accessible and are within your means. You do not need to include specific foods or avoid foods. A good meal plan is one that will provide you with all the nutrients that you need.

Calculate how many calories you need

To lose weight, you need to consume calories a little less than what your body needs to maintain current body weight. You should not restrict your calorie intake too much. Rapid weight loss means that you lost excessive lean tissue and your metabolism will slow down. A rapid weight gain can also follow.

Calculate your total energy allowance and deduct 500 calories. This can result in weight loss of 1 pound per week. And if you increase your physical activities, you can have a total weight loss of 2 pounds per week. This rate supports fat loss and retains lean tissue.

Focus on the nutrients you can get

Meeting your energy needs is hard when you are having fewer calories in a day. So, make sure to choose foods that will provide you the most nutrients. Your diet must emphasize vegetables, fruits, lean meats or alternatives, whole grains and low-fat milk products.

Eat smaller meals

Eat small portions of food at each meal. You do not need to skip any meals. Just remember to eat enough food that will provide you with sufficient energy, vitamins, minerals and some satisfaction.

Choose lower energy-dense food

There are foods that are high in calories but provide you with low satiety, like donuts and chips and there are also foods that are low in calorie but make you feel full for a long time. These foods are high in water and fiber and low in fat. They are also full of vitamins and minerals; they not only support weight loss, but they can also promote good health.

Drink lots of water

Water helps in reducing weight in several ways. For one, foods high in water content increase fullness and reduce hunger. When you drink water before your meal, it will fill your stomach and you will eat less food. Also, if you replace your other beverages with water, you can lower your calorie intake because water has no calories. Water is also helpful for your GI tract to adapt to a high-fiber diet.

Eats foods that are rich in fiber

Foods that are high in fiber are not only low in calories, but they are also high in vitamins and minerals. Fiber can also promote satiety and it means you will eat less.

In addition, you need to put more effort in eating fiber-rich foods because they tend to be harder to chew and swallow, and for this reason, you tend to eat slower. Eating slowly can help you lower your intake of calories.

Choose fat carefully

Fat may not be avoided and it is also good to include in your diet. Just know which fats are beneficial and will not pose danger to your health. Select foods that are rich in monounsaturated fat and polyunsaturated fats. Limit foods that have saturated and trans-fat.

Limit foods with empty calories

To lose weight or maintain good health, a person must watch out not only for fat, but also for sugar and alcohol. Together with your nutrient-dense foods, you can have sugar and alcohol occasionally. But remember, moderation must be observed.

Increase your physical activity

The best way to lose weight is to add physical activities. The more energy you use in physical activities, the more body fat you lose. It is recommended to add a 60 minute moderately intense exercise to your day. This makes your body lose fat faster, keep more muscle and prevents you from regaining weight.

When you exercise, your body expends more calories and can develop more lean tissue. Your body will also have less body fat. Consequently, your metabolic rate will increase. Also, when you exercise you tend to eat less. Your body will use the stored fuels and release glucose and fatty acids in your blood. Because of this, your digestive functions are suppressed.

Exercise can also help you relieve stress and boredom. Stress and boredom often cue inappropriate eating for many but exercise can curb this. In addition, your emotional well-being can also be improved.

Choose activities that you are willing to do regularly. Spend your time doing things more than sitting. Simple things like taking the stairs instead of the elevator, playing outside instead of video games and walking to places instead of using cars, can do wonders for your health.

Be mindful of your environment

Your surroundings, people around you, and other environmental factors greatly influence your eating behavior.

Pay attention to these factors and try to change the factors that you think can help you eat less. Take, for example, when you dine outside with your friends. The duration of a meal is extended because of conversation. With this, you tend to eat more. To avoid this, pace your eating with the person who eats the least and the slowest at the table.

Another environmental factor that can influence your eating habit is the accessibility of food. You will likely eat more food if it is visible or within easy reach. In a study that was conducted, secretaries ate candies that were under their desks and did not eat the candies that were a little farther from them. This shows that you will eat less if the food is not within your easy reach. Therefore, keep non-nutritious foods, especially junk foods, out of sight and out of your mind. Stock your fridge or pantry with foods that are low in calories and keep the high-calorie ones away.

Portion sizes of foods can also affect your diet. These days, foods are packed in big sizes and you will most likely eat them all. To avoid overeating, you can repack foods into smaller portions or eat them off a plate. Select plates, bowls, and glasses that are smaller in size to create illusions of eating a big portion of food.

Change your behavior and attitude

Your behavior and attitude towards achieving your goals are big influences to be successful. Prepare yourself for the changes that will happen to increase your energy expenditure and decrease calorie intake. You need to be determined and focused. Also, adopt a positive outlook and make sure to not think of your strategies as temporary. Make them a part of your daily life to maintain a healthy body.

It is good to have a reflection on oneself to be able to determine the eating habits that need to be addressed. Also, list the physical activities you have. With this record, you have a base that can help you with your progress.

With your unwanted behaviors written down, examine why that behavior happened and think of ways to prevent them from happening. For example, you overeat whenever you are stressed. Focus on what you want to happen and try to change gradually. You can start on small things and try a reward system to support your efforts.

Successful weight loss strategies need a strong mind to identify the problems and find ways to respond to them appropriately. And of course, it will be better if you have emotional support from the people around you to help you cope with the changes you are making.

Calorie in vs. calorie out

The key to an effective weight management is to control your calories. By eating food, nutritious and not-so-nutritious food alike, you fuel yourself with calories. This is calories in. Now, the body needs to use calories as energy in order to function. When the body uses such calories, then it can be referred to as calories out.

Whether your aim is to gain or lose weight, it all depends on how you manage your calories (calorie in vs. calorie out). If you want to gain weight, which is essential if you want to build more muscle mass, then you should be on a calorie surplus. This means that you should consume more calories than the number of calories that your body uses. This simply means that you need to eat more. However, if your goal is to lose weight, then you should be on a calorie deficit. This means that you should eat less than the calories that your body uses. Simply put, it means that you should eat less.

Intermittent Fasting

This type of fasting is popular these days. As the name suggests, you observe a cycle for fasting and eating. For example, you eat within an 8-hour window and fast during the remaining 16 hours. Some would eat within a shorter time period, such as 6 hours or even less, and then spend the other hours fasting. This kind of eating habit tends to make you consume fewer calories than normal, which naturally results in weight loss.

Do not be afraid of fasting. In fact, the human body is well designed for fasting. Our ancestors had to fast when no food was available which occurred often. Fasting is normal, even Jesus fasted in the desert for 40 days; other people have fasted for longer periods. And, take note that this is only intermittent fasting, which means that you will still eat. Therefore, this is easier and more doable.

The most common kind of intermittent fasting is the 16/8 method where you fast for 16 hours and eat within the remaining time of 8 hours. This may also involve skipping breakfast.

Another method is the eat-stop-eat method. This is for those who are already used to intermittent fasting; hence, not for beginners. By using this method, you should fast for 24 hours about once or even twice a week.

The 5:2 intermittent fasting diet is also common. This simply means eating very little, about 500 calories for two consecutive days. You can then eat normally during the other 5 remaining days.

There are many other ways to apply intermittent fasting. The key is to have a cycle for fasting and eating. Of course, if you are serious about losing weight, you should also be mindful of what you eat during an eating cycle.

Flexible dieting and IIFYM approach can be applied with intermittent fasting. In fact, intermittent fasting can significantly improve the effects of this diet. If properly observed and matched up with regular exercise, it is guaranteed that you will lose that stubborn fat and have a better-looking physique.

Fasting vs. starvation

It is worth noting that fasting is not the same as starvation. Starvation is involuntary, marked with the absence of food, while fasting is a voluntary act where you do not eat even when there is food on the table. Fasting is also usually resorted to for physical, mental, and even spiritual purposes. Although starvation and fasting are characterized by not eating, they have different reasons, intentions and purposes.

How to break a fast

Simply put, you break a fast by eating. Take, for example, the term "breakfast," it signifies that you break a fast by eating. However, what to eat and how much you should eat also matter. This is true, especially if you are not yet used to fasting. The way to break a fast depends on how long you fast. A good thing to remember is that you should break the fast gently. Do not break a fast by eating a large meal. Doing so might give you a bad stomach ache. A good way to break a fast is by drinking fresh juice, eating soup or some salad. However, if you have only fast for several hours, then breaking a fast will not be a problem. Any light meal will do. The more you get used to intermittent fasting, the easier it will be for you to break a fast.

Do not fast

As a rule, anybody can do intermittent fasting. However, there are a few instances when you should not engage in any kind of fasting, such as when you are below 18 years of age. This is because your body needs all the nutrients that it can get. After all, such an age is too young for any form of fasting. There is simply no need for it. Another instance is when you are pregnant or breastfeeding. This is because you need to have enough nutrients to share with your child. Another circumstance where you should not engage in any form of fasting is when you are underweight or when your BMI is less than 18.5.

Effects of intermittent fasting

Fasting is not just about taking in fewer calories. It goes much further than that. In fact, it has remarkable effects on the body. It affects the body deeply, all the way down to the molecular level.

Human Growth Hormone (HGH)

Fasting can increase your HGH by about five times over. This usually results in significant fat loss and even muscle gain, among other things.

Cell repair

When you reach the state of fasting, the cells undergo their repair processes. This also includes the removal of dysfunctional proteins that are inside cells. As can be imagined, such cell repair is highly beneficial to the body.

Lowers insulin level

The level of insulin drops when you are in a fasting state. A lower level of insulin means that your fat reserves can easily be tapped and used as energy.

Genes

When in a fasting state, your gene functions enhance so you can enjoy other health benefits, as well as protection from other diseases. You can also enjoy longevity.

Take note that the above are just some of the notable benefits on a cellular level. Other benefits to the body, such as weight loss, better skin and others, are also a part of the expected benefits of intermittent fasting.

Health benefits of intermittent fasting

Now that you know the benefits of intermittent fasting on a molecular level, it is time for you to know other remarkable benefits of intermittent fasting, which are directly related to your overall health.

Weight loss

Obviously, weight loss is a natural effect of intermittent fasting. It is an effective way to stave off that stubborn belly fat and be fit and healthy. Moreover, since there is a period of eating, you will not feel so deprived of the foods that you love to eat.

Heart benefits

This type of fasting effectively lowers LDL cholesterol, insulin resistance and triglycerides, among others. These are the factors that increase your heart risk.

Anti-aging

Intermittent fasting is the way to longevity. It is also known to extend the lifespan of rats. And, since it triggers the cellular repair process, you can also enjoy younger-looking skin.

Prevents cancer

Various studies show that intermittent fasting can help reduce the risk of cancer.

Beneficial to the brain

Intermittent fasting triggers the brain hormone, BDNF, which can aid in the production of new nerve cells. It can also help prevent Alzheimer's disease.

Insulin resistance

Intermittent fasting is popular as an effective method to decrease insulin levels and blood sugar. If you have problems with type 2 diabetes, then you may find intermittent fasting a great help.

There are other health benefits of intermittent fasting as well. This type of fasting is so amazing that many people want to try it. Of course, if it is your first time to fast, you may encounter some challenges, such as headaches, nausea, mood swings, and others; but such are only temporary. Once your body has adapted to these types of eating habits, then you can enjoy the remarkable benefits that it offers.

On safety

One of the things that people ask about intermittent fasting is if it is safe or not. To put simply, intermittent fasting is safe as long as you do it properly. Do not aim for quick developments. Just aim for a gradual progress — slow, yet safe and sure. Do not fast for 24 hours if it is your first time doing intermittent fasting.

What to expect

Hunger — anything that is related to fasting is marked with hunger. You should realize that hunger is just like a wave in an ocean. It comes and goes. It does not stay. When you feel hungry during a fasting cycle, do not feed the hunger by focusing on it. Instead, do something fun or get busy with something else. For beginners, you may find hunger hard to deal with. However, as your body adapts to this eating habit, you will find hunger easier to manage. In fact, you might not feel hungry anymore.

You may also feel your body getting weak, some headaches and mood swings. These are natural effects when one is hungry. Just stay strong and allow your body to adjust. Once your body has adjusted to intermittent fasting, you will feel energized and also enjoy the many benefits of intermittent fasting. How long your body takes to adjust may vary, but it may take a few days to a few weeks.

Take note that during a fasting cycle, you can still drink water, tea, and coffee. Just stick to no calorie or very low-calorie tea or coffee. It is good to drink coffee because it can make you feel satiated. In fact, it can trick you into feeling full even when you are fasting.

You can also engage in physical activities even when fasting. Hence, you can still do your workout and other exercises during a fasting cycle. If it is your first time to fast, then you might want to just do some light exercises, like jogging. However, once your body has adjusted to the eating habit of intermittent fasting, you will feel much stronger and be able to do intense exercises without any problem, even when on a fasting cycle. It may take time for your body to get used to intermittent fasting, but it is well worth the time and effort that you put in.

Chapter 3: Fad Diets

It is good to have an understanding of fad diets so that you will not be victim of such spurious diet programs, as well as be able to identify genuine diet programs such as the Flexible Diet with IIFYM approach. Here are some notable features that characterize fad diets:

Dramatic weight loss

Most fad diets promote dramatic weight loss in a short period of time. A healthy diet, such as the Flexible Diet, also promotes weight loss, but it does so gradually. Rapid weight loss is usually due to mere loss of water or is a mere temporary fix. The lost weight is quickly restored the moment you rehydrate yourself with lots of water or when you start eating normally.

Poor nutrition

Although many of these fad diets will make you lose weight quickly, you can expect to end up with a weak body due to poor nutrition. A good and healthy diet must not deprive you of the needed calories for your body to function properly. Your body also needs a steady supply of macronutrients, as well as an assortment of minerals and vitamins, among others.

Relying on liquid formulas

Many of the fad diets rely heavily on liquid formulas. A truly healthy diet does not depend solely on liquid formulas. To have a healthy body, you need to eat real and solid foods. Although liquids, such as water, are essential to health, solid foods are also equally important.

Relying on special foods and devices

Fad diets may require you to eat some special food or use a special device, while a healthy diet relies on fresh and nutritious foods. A good diet will teach you to make good choices from the conventional food supply, and not depend on any artificial or special food. After all, the more natural and fresh the food is, the better.

Do not teach to live healthily

Many of these fad diets only lay down a set of rules to follow and do not teach you to live healthily. A good and healthy diet will encourage you to change your lifestyle into something that is healthier. Hence, even when not on a diet, you get to make healthy choices and also live clean and healthy.

Collect a huge amount of money

Some of these fad diets will ask for a huge amount of deposit before you can learn their secrets. Take note that a payment may be considered okay provided it is reasonably priced and on a pay-as-you-go basis. However, when the amount is too much, or if there is nothing to back up the program's claims except the testimony of the seller or some fake testimonials, then beware because it might be a sign that you are dealing with a scammer who just wants to rip you off.

They fail to educate people

All of these fad diets are so focused on themselves that they fail to educate their clients on what it really means to be healthy. Also, instead of promoting spurious weight-loss tips and tricks, they should strive to teach their clients to focus on nutrient-rich foods and encourage their clients to exercise regularly.

Lack of any post-diet program

Fad diets usually do not express any concern for their clients in that they do not provide any weight maintenance program after the diet or after achieving your fitness goals. A healthy diet will not leave you unaided, but will provide helpful guidelines and information on what to do even after achieving your fitness objectives.

Examples of fad diets

Here are some remarkable examples of fad diets. Take note that some of these fad diets are still being promoted even today:

High-protein diet

As the name implies, this diet is characterized by eating large amounts of protein in order to lose weight, as well as to build muscles. This is a fad because muscles do not just come from protein. The key to building muscles is exercise, or more specifically, resistance training. And, although you need protein to build more muscles, you do not need any excess protein. In fact, consuming too much protein is risky and dangerous. This kind of diet puts too much stress on the kidneys and liver. Also, excess protein usually turns into fat.

Liquid diet

A liquid diet relies on only consuming liquids and staying away from solid foods. The problem with this diet is that you do not get all the nutrients that your body needs. For example, some essential nutrients like phytochemicals can only come from eating fruits and vegetables. Another noticeable disadvantage of a liquid diet is that you quickly recover the lost pounds once you return to eating solid food. This fad diet does offer a quick fix for weight loss, but it is only temporary.

Pure cabbage diet

As the name implies, this is a diet primarily of cabbage. So, you eat nothing but cabbage. This is a fad diet because this only makes you shed off water weight and not excess fat. Therefore, you can rest assured that you will experience an increase in your weight once you return to your regular eating habit. Another disadvantage of this diet program is that it fails to supply the body with the nutrition that it needs in order to function properly. Like other fad diets, you cannot use this diet for long periods of time without any undesirable consequences.

Grapefruit diet

Similar to a cabbage diet, the grapefruit diet is about eating only grapefruit and nothing else. The problem with such single-food diet programs is that they fail to give the body the right nourishment that it needs. Such fad diets are simply too restrictive and miss out on other needed nutrients, vitamins and minerals.

Juice diet

Again, for the same reasons as aforesaid, this diet is also not good for your body. Take note that you do not just need a diet that will make you lose weight; you need a diet that is healthy for your body. After all, if losing weight is your only concern, the best way is simply not to eat anything. But, a good diet means much more than losing weight. It is about being healthy and making healthy choices.

Long fasts

If done for a spiritual purpose, then there is nothing wrong with this. In fact, Jesus fasted in the desert for 40 days without food and water. Needless to say, long fasting will make you lose weight effectively. However, fasting for a long period of time also tends to lower your metabolism. The problem here is that once you resume your regular eating habit, you can easily regain the weight that you have lost. Also, this kind of diet (if you should refer to it as a diet) is not permanent, and it does not teach you how to be healthy.

Common problems with fad diets

Here are some notable problems that you will have to deal with when you engage in a fad diet:

Temporary weight loss

The quick-fix offer of fad diets is very tempting to accept. However, the problem with such offers is that the weight loss that you achieve will be hard to maintain. This is true, especially if the weight loss is merely due to the decrease in water weight, which is a common thing in fad diets.

Increased risk of diseases

Since many fad diets will deprive you of foods which, in turn, will deprive you of essential nutrients that the body needs, you expose yourself to many risks and diseases. Take, for example, the famous high-protein diet. Such diet can increase the loss of calcium, which exposes you to osteoporosis. A diet that is high in protein and low in carbs can also trigger calcium oxalate and uric acid to form, which can be the cause of kidney stones.

Reduced physical performance

It should be noted that a healthy diet should make your body healthy and not weak. Fad diets are known for reducing your physical performance. This is because such diets usually place a serious restriction on your carbohydrate intake. When you do not consume enough carbs, the body uses its fluids and electrolytes. When these, too, are used up, it can cause a dramatic drop in blood pressure and physical or athletic performance.

Ketosis

It is worth noting that being in a state of ketosis is not completely bad. However, if left unmanaged, you can expect some serious and unpleasant consequences. This state is often reached when one is in starvation mode for a long period. Although this may seem natural, this is the state where the body struggles to survive. One of the signs that you have entered ketosis is the keto breath. Keto breath is usually defined as a fruity scent or smell to your breath. Although described as something "fruity," it is not really that pleasant to have.

Gain more weight

Some of these fad diets will make you lose weight, but then trigger you to gain more weight after the diet. This is because many of these quick-fix diets depend on making you eat too little. Hence, once you return to your normal eating habit and eat more food as a way to reward yourself, you quickly add on new pounds. And since such fad diets do not really teach you to value being healthy, you will find it easy and natural to gain more weight since you are not a healthy person yourself.

Can fad diets make you lose weight?

Yes, fad diets can make you lose weight. In fact, they can make you lose lots of weight. And, if you know how to return to your regular eating habits without ruining the benefits that you have received from your diet, including fad diets, then you can still take advantage of such fad diets. However, the problem with fad diets is that you do not become healthy. Yes, you lose weight, but that is about all. You do not learn to be healthy and make healthy decisions or change your preferences. Once you are back to your regular eating habit, you will then easily regain whatever weight you have lost, simply because you are back to not being healthy. Hence, any weight loss that you achieve through fad diets is only temporary.

A truly healthy diet will make you healthy. Therefore, even if you return to your regular eating habit, you will not have to worry about gaining back any weight that you have lost. A good and effective diet like the Flexible Diet will teach you more than losing weight. It will encourage you to live a healthier lifestyle and be truly healthy yourself. In a way, it changes a person in a positive light.

Chapter 4: Exercises

You can add in regular exercise to increase the deficit and speed up weight loss. Exercise also develops the muscles, which will give you that well-shaped and stunning physique that you have always wanted. Since Flexible Dieting is not a strict diet and will give you enough energy, you can engage in high intensity workouts. Now, there are many exercises that you can do. In fact, you do not even have to go to the gym just to break some serious sweat.

Depending on your physical level of fitness, you can do light and/or high intensity workout training. To be safe, you may want to visit your doctor to know if you can safely engage in a strenuous physical activity. Do not worry; even if you cannot do high intensity workouts, you can still do some low intensity exercises to keep fit and lose more weight.

As you may already know, a healthy diet and regular exercise are the keys to being healthy and fit. If you think that a high intensity workout is difficult for you, you can start with a light exercise such as walking or jogging, and slowly build your way up from there.

Walking for weight loss

Walking is one of the best and most effective ways to shred some fat. A study in Britain shows that people who regularly engage in a walking exercise tend to weigh less than those engaged in other forms of exercises. This is because walking is a light form exercise. You can do it anytime and as much as you want. In fact, it is the kind of exercise that you can do safely even every day.

Many people have lost weight simply by walking on a regular basis. Depending on your current physical level and the intensity of your walk, you can expect to lose from a half-pound up to 2 pounds every week.

Although walking is an activity that is open to everyone and is safe to do, you may want to visit your doctor first to ensure that such physical activity is safe for your body. Of course, this is only recommended if you have some physical issues or problems. After all, walking can be a taxing activity, especially if you engage in long, brisk walks.

Walking is a safe activity and exercise. However, if you start to feel uncomfortable, or if you feel nauseous or any pain, this is a sign that you should stop for a while and take a break. When you engage in any physical activity, regardless of how light it is, you should learn to listen to your body. Remember that walking should be a light activity. So, enjoy every walk, and avoid too much exertion, especially if you want to do this long term.

Jogging

If you want to improve your stamina and endurance, you should hit the road or the treadmill. Jogging is also a very effective exercise for losing weight. You can also adjust the intensity of this exercise by changing your speed.

It is ideal to jog outside and enjoy nature. However, if this is not possible, or if you live in a city that is highly polluted, then you can jog on a treadmill or simply in place.

For a start, you can try to jog for 15 minutes. You can also alternate jogging and walking, so as to give you time to catch your breath. Jogging is a light form of exercise. Advice given by professionals is this: If you cannot carry on a conversation while jogging, then you should lower the speed of your jog. Do not worry; your speed will develop once your body gets used to jogging.

Jogging in place is also an excellent option. You can jog in place while you enjoy your favorite movie. Although jogging in place is easier than jogging outside, you can increase the intensity of the exercise by lifting your knees higher and adding some quick jumping jacks.

Jogging on a regular basis is an excellent way to lose weight. The best time to walk or jog depends on your personal schedule. While some people can exercise every morning, others have a busy schedule and can only workout in the evening. Regardless of the time when you can exercise, the important thing is to make time for it, be it in the morning, afternoon or even before going to bed. Although jogging can be fun, you should give your body, especially your legs and knees, enough time to rest.

High intensity bodyweight workout

The best way to exercise for weight loss is by doing high intensity exercises. Such exercises can get your heart pumping at an increased rate, which translates to higher calorie consumption and fat burn. Take note that the more effort that you put into your workout, the more calories and fat you can burn.

There is no need for you to engage in some intense workout, but if you are looking forward to burning a serious amount of fat within a short period of time, then high intensity interval training (HIIT) is the one for you. As the name suggests, this kind of workout is composed of short periods of rest and high intensity exercises. If your fitness level is not yet ready for such intense workout, you may adjust the intensity by doing fewer reps or simply decreasing the speed of the exercises. The important thing is to put in more effort and get your heart pumping.

The workout

Killer 55

This exercise is very effective in developing your arm and leg muscles. It is also effective in increasing your heart rate. The way to do this is by doing 5 squats followed by 5 pushups. For a start, just do the regular squats and pushups.

A set of 5 squats followed by 5 pushups constitutes 1 set. Do this for 10 sets continuously. Again, you can lower the intensity of your workout if you find it too difficult for you.

Once you get used to this workout, you can then use one-legged squats followed by a one-arm pushup. You can also increase the number of sets and reps per set.

High knees to burpees

Burpees is one of the most popular bodyweight exercises. They really test your endurance, especially if you do them for a long period. You can further enhance this exercise by combining it with another taxing exercise, such as the high knees stationary jogging.

The way to do this exercise is to do jog in place, but keep your knees high. This will demand more effort on your part and will result in more calorie and fat burn. Do this for 10 seconds, and then immediately do burpees for another 10 seconds. This is one set, which takes only 20 seconds to complete. Try to do 10 sets of this exercise.

Jumping jacks to mountain climbers

Everybody knows how fun doing jumping jacks can be. Well, jumping jacks are also effective in burning fat. Mountain climbers are also effective not only in increasing your heart rate, but also in developing the abs and arm muscles.

For this exercise, you should do 10 seconds of jumping jacks at a fast pace, and then follow them up with 10 seconds of mountain climbers. If this is easy for you, you may increase the intensity of the exercise by increasing your speed. Try to do 20 sets without any rest.

Sprint and push up

It is good to do this exercise in an open space. If you do not have an open space, you can simply run in place. Just be sure to lift your knees high and quickly to add more intensity to your workout. So, the way to do this exercise is simply to sprint as fast as you can for 10 seconds and then do 10 pushups. This is 1 set. Try to do 5 to 10 sets. Once you get used to this workout, you can increase the time and the number of sets.

Punching bag

Using a punching bag is not only fat burning, it is also an excellent way to increase your heart rate and release serious energy and sweat. Punch the bag for 3 minutes, and then rest for 1 minute. Try to use different punches and combinations. Also, be sure to hit the bag with a series of punches. Do not focus on the strength or power behind every punch. Instead, focus on executing the punches smoothly and quickly. Once you get used to the movement, you can then start adding power and strength. A good combination to start with is the jab-jab-cross combination. Be sure to maintain proper form, and do not forget to breathe.

SPP

SPP stands for Squat, Plank, Pushup exercise routine. To do this, you should squat down. Instead of returning to a standing position, you should place your hands on the floor, and then kick back your legs and assume a full plank position. You then execute a pushup. After which, immediately jump your legs back into a squat position, and then repeat. Adjust the number of sets according to your fitness level. Do not forget to tighten your abs as you go through the movements.

Jumping squats

This is a combination of jumping jacks and squats. The way to do this is to squat down; and, instead of pushing your way back up to the standing position, you should perform a jumping jack, which will bring you into a standing position where you can execute another squat. Try to do as many reps as you can.

Modified sit-ups

Sit-ups may be boring for some, but you can increase the intensity of your sit-ups to make the exercise more challenging. A good way to do this is by lifting your legs as you go through the movements of a regular sit-up. The higher you lift your legs, the hard the exercise will be. Also, be sure to keep your legs straight, and do not let your head touch the ground.

Jumping jacks + clapping pushups

Perform 5 quick jumping jacks, and then follow up with 2 clapping pushups. Make sure to do the moves smoothly. You may also increase the number of reps as you progress.

Run-walk

This is a common exercise yet very effective way to lose weight. Simply alternate running and walking. It is good to do this outside, so you will have a big space to run. However, if it is raining or if running outside would not be a good choice, you may simply use a treadmill or just run in place.

When you walk, try to do brisk walking by simply walking at a faster pace. This will allow you to burn more calories. Of course, the speed by which you execute this exercise depends on your level of physical fitness. Feel free to adjust the intensity of the exercise according to your preference.

Pullup-squats

If you have a place where you can do a pull-up, then you might find this exercise interesting. Pull-ups are good for your upper body, especially for your biceps and shoulders, while squats are excellent for your lower body.

As the name already implies, simply do as many pull-ups as you can, and then follow up with as many squats as you can. These two successive movements compose 1 set. Do as many sets as you can.

Try YouTube

YouTube has many exercise channels. These videos will show you interesting bodyweight HIIT cardio exercises that will help you burn lots of calories. Do as many exercises as you can.

Be creative

Be creative and develop your own routine and exercise. There is really no wrong way to do this. Learn to listen to your body, and you will know which exercises are good for you. Feel free to combine the exercises in this book with other exercises that you know. The key is to keep on moving. The more you move and the more pressure you apply to yourself, the more calories you will burn. Keep your heart rate up and never stop moving. Of course, you are free to take short breaks, but be sure to get back to the exercises quickly.

Everyday activities

You do not always need to be at the gym or your home gym just to shred off some calories and fat. After all, your body is always in a state where you use up energy from the foods that you eat. Take advantage of everyday activities, such as climbing the stairs instead of using the elevator when you go to malls. Another good practice is to park your car farther than the usual from the entrance door. This will not only give you a big space to park your car, but will also give you an opportunity to enjoy a good walk and burn more calories.

If you spend lots of time on the computer, you might want to request a stand-up table, so you can use the computer while standing. Studies show that you burn twice as many calories when standing than sitting. If you are going to a nearby store, you might want to use your mountain bike or simply walk instead of using your car. Not only will you save money on gas, but it will also give you a good opportunity to exercise.

Simple everyday activities can be turned into something meaningful and effective for your fitness goals. Do not be lazy but enjoy every moment that presents itself. Being healthy is a choice, and it is a way of life.

Chapter 5: Keys to Success

These keys to success constitute the best practices that you should observe so that you will get good results from your diet and exercise. It is important that you apply these tips and live with them because they are the best practices that will help give you the fit and healthy body you have always dreamed of.

Stick to your diet

Flexible Dieting has long been proven to be effective in sculpting a body that you can be proud of. It will give you a body that is both healthy and fit. However, to enjoy the benefits of this diet, you should stick to it.

Even before you begin dieting, you should already expect to encounter some challenges and strong temptations. These are temptations that will lead you to abandon your diet, which means giving up on your fitness goals. Being tempted to give up is normal, but actually giving up by abandoning your diet program is wrong. Fortunately, Flexible Dieting is not like other diet plans that are very strict. Flexible Dieting allows you to enjoy even your favorite junk foods from time to time. Just remember that every time you feel like giving up, simply stop thinking and stick to your diet.

Keeping a fitness journal

Although not required, writing a fitness journal can be very helpful. Do not worry; you do not need to be a professional writer to have your own fitness journal. The important thing is simply for you to write honestly and update your journal regularly.

Ideally, your fitness journal should include the reasons why you want to be on a diet. You should also write down your fitness goals, your current fitness level, and the objectives that you want to accomplish in the long run. During the times that you are tempted to abandon your diet, you can open your journal and read what you have written to get the inspiration and motivation that you need to continue and remain healthy.

Regular exercise

You can lose more weight by adding exercise to your diet. Exercise is also the only way to develop your muscles and build a stunning physique. After all, merely taking fewer carbs than what you consume is only good for losing weight, but does not give you a toned and well-defined body.

To be healthy and have a good-looking body, you also need to exercise in addition to following a healthy diet, such as the Flexible Diet and IIFM approach. Take note that the exercise should be regular. The key to living healthy is to make diet and exercise a part of your daily life.

Take a break

Take a break. Shredding off that stubborn fat and sculpting a well-defined figure takes time. It can also be very tiring. So, take a break from time to time. Give yourself a chance to just relax. Perhaps drink a glass of fresh juice as you watch a movie. You can also give yourself a cheat meal and treat yourself with some fries, pizzas, and chocolates. After all, such foods are still a part of the Flexible Diet. Learn not to desire anything, accept yourself as you are at the moment, and just relax. Take a break and hit the gym again tomorrow.

Drink lots of water

It is recommended to drink 7-8 glasses of water in a day. Take note, however, that his recommendation is for the average person who does not engage in any strenuous physical activity. This means that the person does not do any running or any HIIT cardio workout. Therefore, you should aim to drink more than 8 glasses of water every day.

Water is important to the body. It cleanses your body and washes the toxins away. It is also good for your skin, as well as for other parts of your body. Drinking water is also a good way to suppress or control your appetite. Most of the time, people confuse hunger for thirst, and end up eating when drinking water would be enough. Make it a habit to have a glass or jug of water with you. What is more, water has zero calories.

Drink coffee

Coffee, especially plain black coffee, has very few calories. Coffee is also a healthy drink, because it is full of antioxidants. What is more, coffee can suppress your appetite. A cup of coffee can make you feel full. Add in a slice of healthy bread, and you will feel satisfied in no time. When you drink coffee, avoid adding white sugar, or at least stick to those that have low calories and sugar content. Research also shows that drinking coffee before you work out is a good way to perform better at the gym (or at home).

Give time for your muscles to recover

It is not recommended to train the same muscle group every day. You should give your muscles enough time to recover. For example, if you do lots of pushups today, let your arms and chest rest the next day. If you really want to exercise, you can just hit a different body part. For example, if your arms are still tired due to the previous day's workout, you can simply do squats and focus on your lower body while your upper body is still recovering. You can also add in some sit-ups if you want.

Cardio exercises are excellent. But, even running can strain your tendons and muscles. This is true, especially when you sprint or do long-distance running. Be sure to always allow your body to recover. After all, there are many different exercises that you can do.

Listen to your body

Whether you are on a diet or busy with a particular workout, listening to your body is a skill that you will always benefit from. By listening to your body, you will know what you need, as well as any adjustments that you should do. Not all bodies are the same, so find out what works for you — and the way to do this is by listening to your body. If a particular exercise makes you feel any pain or even discomfort, then make some adjustments.

Maintain proper form

When you exercise, make sure that you do the exercises with proper form or posture. It is important that you always keep your spine straight. Maintaining proper form is important to avoid injuries, as well as to get the best benefits of an exercise. If you do not know how to execute a particular exercise, you can always ask your gym instructor for instructions. If you love to workout at home, you can always ask a friend to help you. You can also watch some videos on YouTube as to how to execute a certain exercise routine properly.

Have an exercise partner

A good way to enjoy your exercises is to do it with another. You can also invite a good friend to join you on your healthy diet. Just be sure to pick someone who is also serious and interested in living a healthy lifestyle; otherwise, your partner might discourage you instead of giving you more inspiration. It is also nice to talk with your partner about any developments or challenges that you are facing. Before you begin your diet together, make it a point that you should help each other. You must both be committed to attaining your fitness objectives.

An exercise partner can also help you during the times when you feel like giving up. To make it more intimate and interesting, you might want to eat the same food with your partner or even prepare your foods together.

Check the nutrition label

Be sure to check the nutrition label of foods that you buy. Check the count of calories and macronutrients. Check the count per piece or per 100 grams to make it easier to compute. It is best to stay away from junk foods that have a high calorie count. The nutritional label is often found on the back of a food item. It is not displayed on the packaging, you can simply make a search online to track a food's nutritional value.

Choose healthy foods

Make a habit to choose healthy foods over unhealthy ones like junk foods. Unhealthy foods give you a lot of calories with very low nutritional value. Such food also does not make you feel well, especially once you get used to eating healthy foods. Although the Flexible Diet allows you to eat foods that are not nutritious, the consumption of such foods should be limited, and you should strictly observe such limitation.

On having six-pack abs

The much sought for six-pack abs are said to be the holy grail of fitness. It is true that every person has abdominal muscles; however, most do not see them because they are covered with fat. To make the abs visible, you need to shed that fat off of your tummy. To do this, you need to observe a healthy diet and exercise.

Of course, having stunning, six-pack abs is not just about removing that stubborn fat, you also need to develop your abdominal muscles by doing ab exercises, such as sit-ups. It is worth noting that sculpting six-pack abs is not a requirement to enjoy the benefits of having a healthy body.

Have a routine

Getting in a routine may be boring, but not having a routine is more likely to cause a negative outcome. A routine demonstrates discipline. The problem with people who do not have a routine is that they easily come up with excuses to skip their exercises, convinced that they can always exercise some other time.

A routine is only bad when it gets boring. So, spice up your exercise routine with new and exciting exercises. You can find many exercises online. You can also find interesting and creative videos on YouTube. Although there are a few people who do not stick to any routine and still achieve their fitness goals, most people fail to reach any success without any established routine. Without a well-established routine to follow, you need to exercise more discipline. Unfortunately, most people do not have a sufficient amount of discipline to achieve their fitness goals.

Enjoy the healthy feeling

It may take some time before your efforts can be noticeable on a physical level. For example, going for a run will not make you lose pounds in just a single day. In fact, you can expect to look the same after the run just as before you went out to exercise. Although nothing can be seen quickly on a physical level, you can feel and enjoy living a healthy lifestyle. The relaxing and satisfying feeling after a good day's run is simply amazing. Do not worry; the benefit of having a better appearance will come after some time. For now, enjoy your exercises and the pleasant feeling that they give you.

Enjoy a sport

If going to the gym or exercising is something that you do not find interesting, then you can look for a sport that you enjoy playing. Many people do not enjoy lifting weights but are fond of playing basketball or soccer. Such games can be considered excellent exercises that can effectively help you burn calories and fat. The key is to learn to enjoy what you are doing. After all, you are expected to exercise on a regular basis, so you should really have an interest in what you are doing. Boxing is also a good sport that you might want to try. You do not need to limit yourself to a single sport or game. You can try swimming and weightlifting at the same time. Just do what works for you, and stick to the ones that you enjoy.

Take note of the calorie count

When it comes to losing weight, the number of calories that you consume should be your main priority. In fact, Mark Haub, a professor of Human Nutrition in the State of Kansas proved that you can eat unhealthy foods and still achieve a substantial amount of weight loss as long as you are mindful of the calories that you take into your body. Hence, if losing weight is your main fitness goal, then pay close attention to the number of calories that you consume. Take note that to lose weight, you need to have a calorie deficit. This means that you should eat fewer calories than the calories that your body uses. Consequently, if you want to add on some weight, you should be in a calorie surplus. This means that you should consume more calories than the number of calories that your body uses. This is also one of the reasons why you should have the habit of checking the nutritional value of the foods that you eat. Pay attention to the calorie count.

Take advantage of negative calorie foods

Negative calorie foods are foods that have fewer calories than the amount of energy that the body uses to digest them. Hence, eating these foods will naturally result in a caloric deficit, which is the key to weight loss. If you are feeling hungry and afraid of gaining any weight, you can stick to negative calorie foods. Not only will you feel satiated, but you will also burn off calories. Examples of negative calorie foods are apples, lettuce, grapefruit, lemons, celery and cabbage, among others.

Have a long-term plan

This is where many diet programs go wrong. They simply do not have a long-term plan. Once they are able to remove some pounds off of your body, they abandon you without any guidelines to follow. Hence, you simply go back to your normal eating pattern and lifestyle and get the lost pounds back in a few days.

Flexible dieting allows you to have a long-term plan simply because it is a diet that you can safely use for a long-term period. It is also a simple diet with just a few guidelines to observe. Just take in the right amounts of macronutrients and keep your calorie intake to the recommended level for your body. Flexible Dieting with IIFYM approach is very effective and easy to follow.

Dealing with hunger

If you are used to an unhealthy eating habit, you may experience hunger on the first few days that you shift to a healthy diet. Do not worry; this is normal and expected to happen. Unfortunately, hunger can make you feel very uncomfortable. In fact, many people who go on a diet usually fail to stick to their diet because they cannot shake off the uneasy feeling of being hungry. But, fortunately, every feeling of hunger is not permanent. In fact, hunger comes and goes like a wave in the ocean. If you just ignore your hunger and focus on other things, the feeling of hunger will disappear on its own. Also, once you get used to the eating habits of your healthy diet, you will feel less hungry. In fact, just after a week or two, you may no longer feel hungry. After all, when you follow the Flexible Diet with IIFYM approach, you are sure that you do not deprive your body of essential nutrients, especially the macronutrients which are essential to any healthy diet.

Lack of perseverance and discipline

Perseverance and discipline are important for success with any healthy diet program. This is because you cannot see any noticeable changes in just a few days. A true diet takes time to appear on a physical level. However, you can feel its benefits even on the first few days of the diet. If you lack the values of discipline and perseverance, then you might give up the diet even before you start to see any noticeable results. If you are serious about getting fit and healthy, then be sure to have these important values.

Chapter 6: Common Pitfalls

To further guarantee success, you should know the common pitfalls that those who go on a diet face, so that you will be ready for them and not commit the same mistakes. These pitfalls are faced not only by those who engage in Flexible Dieting, but also by those who follow any other diet programs:

Not eating

Just because you want to lose weight does not mean that you should not eat any food. Instead of not eating which will make you feel gloomy and uncomfortable, you should focus on eating healthy foods. Also, not eating will lower your metabolism which is counterproductive to your fitness goals.

Lack of discipline

The most common mistake of those who go on a diet is the lack of discipline to stick to their chosen diet plan. It is easy to ruin your diet with a few slices of pizza in the evening. Fortunately, Flexible Dieting does not deny you the joy of eating this kind of food, but you must keep it under control. This diet does not promote eating junk food anytime you want and as much as you want. Discipline remains important.

Negative thoughts

Stop entertaining negative thoughts. This is true, especially when you are feeling hungry. But, what is a negative thought? Put simply, a negative thought refers to any thought that will lead you to abandon your diet program; for example, an unscheduled cheat meal, or a thought that tells you that you cannot stop eating junk foods and that you simply cannot become fit anymore. These thoughts will never help you live a healthy life, and will only make you add more pounds of stubborn fat to your physique. When you encounter these thoughts, you should change your focus and adopt a more positive mindset. Remember the reasons why you wanted to go on a healthy diet in the first place.

Jerking backwards

If you exercise with weights, then it is important to note that you should avoid jerking backward. Many people usually do this to help them lift a dumbbell or the bar. If you find yourself in such situation, simply lower the amount of weights that you are lifting. It simply means that the current load is too heavy for you. Again, never jerk when you lift weights. Whether you lift weights or use your own bodyweight, you should always perform the movements smoothly, without jerking.

Following fad diets

Fad diets simply get famous due to mere marketing hype. Especially these days when you can spread a word to the whole world with just a click of a mouse, it is easy to promote fad diets. This is one of the reasons why you should have your own understanding of what constitutes a good diet. Just because a particular diet is popular does not always mean that it is effective. Also, unlike the Flexible Diet, not all diet programs can work on everyone.

Not exercising enough

There are people who spend hours exercising but fail to burn a serious number of calories. This is usually because they do not push themselves when they exercise and only remain in their comfort zone. Take note that the muscles will only grow if you put a sufficient amount of stress on it. Also, if a certain routine has become easy for you to do, then increase the intensity of the workout or try an entirely new routine that will compel you to spend more energy and effort. Take note that if a certain workout does not tire or challenge you enough, then you need to make some changes. The time that you spend exercising is not the measure of how effective your workout is; what is important is the quality of your exercises, as well as how well you execute them.

Conclusion

Thanks for making it through to the end of this book. We hope it was informative and able to provide you with all of the tools that you need to achieve your goals whatever they may be.

The next step is to apply everything that you have learned. So, apply the Flexible Diet and IIFYM approach, and start working on that fit and healthy body that you have always dreamed of.

Finally, if you found this book useful in any way, a review on Amazon is always appreciated!

About The Book

Flexible Dieting & IIFYM: How to Burn Fat & Build Muscle by Eating Your Favorite Foods is your one-stop guide to everything that you need to know about Flexible Dieting and IIFYM (If It Fits Your Macros). Stay away from fad diets and only stick to the one that always works. This book is your handy manual that will teach you:

- The basics of Flexible Dieting with IIFYM approach
- The importance of macronutrients
- How to calculate the right number of calories for your body
- Intermittent fasting
- Effective exercises that can help you lose weight and sculpt a better physique
- The best practices of any successful diet programs
- The common pitfalls and how you can avoid them

And so much more!

This book is the holy grail that will teach you the best way to lose weight and be fit and healthy. *NOW* is the time to make a change and live a happier life. If you want to have a body that is healthy and strong, a body that you can be proud of, then this book is for you.